BALANCING HORMONES FOR WEIGHT LOSS FOR WOMEN

A Concise Guide for Women to Lose Weight through Hormone Harmony

James Edwards

TABLE OF CONTENTS

INTRODUCTION

CHAPTER ONE

The Effect of Estrogen Hormone on Weight Control

CHAPTER TWO

The Effect of Insulin Hormone on Weight Control

CHAPTER THREE

The Effect of Thyroid Hormones on Weight Control

CHAPTER FOUR

The Effect of Nutrition on Hormone Balance for Weight Loss

CHAPTER FIVE

The Influence of Exercise on Hormone Balance for Weight Loss

CHAPTER SIX

Enhancing Hormone Harmony for Weight Loss by Controlling Stress

CHAPTER SEVEN

Utilizing Herbal Remedies for Balancing Hormones for Weight Loss

CHAPTER EIGHT

Mastering Hormone Replacement Therapy For Weight Loss

CONCLUSION

ABOUT THE AUTHOR

INTRODUCTION

This book offers a thorough explanation of the complex connection between hormones and controlling weight. It's critical to learn more about the science underlying how hormones affect our bodies in the modern world, when wellness and health are of utmost importance, especially for women who are struggling with weight reduction.

We'll study the intricacies of hormones and how they affect weight reduction. Gaining knowledge about the functions of insulin, cortisol, thyroid hormones, and sex hormones like progesterone and estrogen as well as how these hormones work closely with one another will help you greatly comprehend the biological processes underlying weight fluctuations.

We'll investigate how hormones are essential to your body's capacity to regulate weight. Hormones are potent transmitters that can help or impede your weight loss objective. They control metabolic rate, hunger, and fat dispersion and storage in the body. Comprehending these mechanisms is essential to formulating a customized strategy to accomplish enduring weight control objectives.

We'll talk about the typical hormonal abnormalities that cause women to acquire weight. We'll examine how hormone imbalances caused by illnesses like polycystic ovary syndrome, thyroid issues, stress, and menopause affect hormone levels and how they might make it difficult to keep a healthy weight by upsetting the body's natural balance.

You'll discover practical tactics, useful advice, and professional insights all in this book to guide you over the challenges of hormone balance for losing weight successfully. Notwithstanding if you're looking to conquer particular hormonal difficulties or are just beginning your effort to a healthy lifestyle, this book will provide you with the information and resources you need to experience long-lasting improvements.

Are you prepared to discover the methods of hormone-driven weight control? Together, let's go on this fascinating adventure to learn how hormones can be used to improve your health and overall comfort.

CHAPTER ONE

The Effect of Estrogen Hormone on Weight Control

A very important hormone in the body, estrogen is most recognized for its ability to control women's menstrual cycles and reproductive processes. Its impact, however, goes well beyond reproduction and is important for metabolism, body structure, and weight control. We will examine the connection between estrogen and body weight in this chapter, as well as the idea of estrogen dominance and how it affects the accumulation of weight. Additionally, we will go over methods for naturally regulating estrogen levels to promote good weight control.

Estradiol, estrone, and estriol are the hormones that make up the group known as estrogen. Although tiny amounts are also formed in the adrenal glands and adipose tissues, women's ovaries are the primary site of production for these hormones. It follows that only a very small quantity of estrogen is found in men, which is produced by the testes and the adrenal glands.

Four Basic Functions of Estrogen Hormone in the Body

1. Menstrual cycle regulation: By promoting the growth of the uterine lining in the follicular phase of menstruation, estrogen aids in the control of the menstrual cycle.

2. Bone health: Osteoporosis prevention and bone density preservation are greatly aided by estrogen.

3. Reproductive health: The growth of secondary sexual traits in women, such as breast size and body fat dissemination, depends on estrogen.

4. Metabolism: Insulin responsiveness, fat storage, and energy exertion are all controlled by estrogen.

Understanding Estrogen Dominance and Its Relationship to Weight Gain

A lack of harmony in the ratio of estrogen to other hormones, like progesterone, is referred to as estrogen dominance. Although many physiological processes require estrogen, an overabundance of estrogen or a relative lack of progesterone can result in adverse changes in hormone harmony that exacerbate weight gain and other health-related problems.

The Four Fundamental Causes of Estrogen Dominance

1. Excessive body fat: People who are obese have greater estrogen levels because fat cells, particularly those in the abdomen, have the capacity to make and store estrogen.

2. Environmental toxins: Some environmental pollutants can mimic estrogen in the body and lead to estrogen dominance. Examples of these pollutants are xenoestrogens, which are found in plastics, insecticides, and personal care items.

3. Hormonal birth control: Certain hormonal birth control methods, especially those that use synthetic estrogen, have the potential to upset the body's natural hormone harmony and promote estrogen dominance.

4. Stress: Prolonged stress can interfere with the metabolism and synthesis of hormones, causing a lack of harmony that results in estrogen dominance.

Four Possible Ways in Which an Individual's Body Weight May Be Affected by Estrogen Dominance

1. Increased fat storage: Excessive estrogen levels, especially in the abdomen, might encourage fat storage, especially when combined with insulin resistance.

2. Water retention: Water retention brought on by estrogen might result in swelling out and momentary weight gain.

3. Slowed metabolism: A lack of harmony in progesterone and estrogen can impact energy exertion and metabolic rate, making weight loss more difficult.

4. Control of Appetite: Our appetite is controlled by estrogen, so a lack of harmony in estrogen could result in an increased appetite and cravings, particularly for foods heavy in fat and sugar.

Six Strategies for Balancing Estrogen Levels Naturally

Establishing perfect harmony in estrogen levels within the body is critical for general health and successful weight control. Here are six methods to help maintain normal estrogen levels:

1. Balanced Diet: Consume a diet that is well-balanced and rich in whole foods, such as fruits, vegetables, lean meats, and healthy fats. Incorporate foods high in

phytoestrogens, such as legumes, soybeans, and flaxseeds, which can assist in controlling estrogen levels.

2. Control Stress: To establish proper hormone harmony, engage in stress-reduction practices like yoga, deep breathing exercises, meditation, or spending time in beautiful natural places like beaches and gardens.

3. Keep your weight in check: A balanced diet and frequent exercise should be combined to help you maintain a healthy weight. One factor that can lead to estrogen dominance is excess body fat.

4. Reduce exposure to toxins: Choose organic produce, use chemical-free cleaning and personal care products, stay away from plastics containing bisphenol-A and other dangerous chemicals, and reduce your exposure to environmental pollutants.

5. Promote the health of your liver: The liver is essential for the metabolization and excretion of hormones, including estrogen. Eat foods high in cruciferous vegetables (broccoli, kale, Brussels sprouts) to aid liver function; these veggies have chemicals that assist in the purification of hormones.

6. Take into account herbal supplements: Black cohosh, dong quai, and chaste berry (Vitex agnus-castus) are a few herbs that have been generally used to improve women's hormonal balance. Before beginning any herbal supplementation regimen, it's important that you seek professional counsel.

Finally, it should be noted that estrogen has a variety of intricate functions in the body, including controlling body weight. Weight gain and metabolic problems can be caused by estrogen dominance, which is defined as a lack of harmony in estrogen levels compared to other hormones. People can promote proper estrogen levels, enhance general health, and control their weight by implementing healthy lifestyle practices, such as eating a balanced diet, managing their stress, exercising frequently, and using natural therapies. Seeking advice from a medical professional or hormone specialist may also offer tailored direction and assistance in properly managing hormone abnormalities.

CHAPTER TWO

The Effect of Insulin Hormone on Weight Control

Among several hormones in the body, insulin plays a major function in controlling blood sugar levels. Anyone trying to achieve hormone harmony for weight loss must understand how insulin functions and how it relates to weight control.

Understanding the Relationship Between Insulin and Body Weight

The pancreas secretes the hormone insulin, which enables your body to either store glucose from carbohydrates in food for later use or utilize the glucose for the production of energy. A meal high in carbohydrates causes an increase in blood sugar levels. In reaction, the pancreas secretes insulin to facilitate the uptake of glucose into cells for energy production.

The modern diet, which is high in processed foods and refined sugars, can cause an imbalance in the insulin system. Repeated releases of insulin from persistent blood sugar rises can eventually cause cells to become desensitized to the influence of insulin. Insulin resistance is an issue that is common to metabolic illnesses such as type 2 diabetes and is strongly associated with unduly addition of weight.

Three Major Ways Insulin Hormone Affects Body Weight

1. Energy Storage: Insulin encourages the liver and muscles to store extra glucose as glycogen. The body turns the leftover glucose into fat for prolonged energy storage when these glycogen stores are congested.

2. Fat Storage: Elevated insulin levels prevent the disintegration of stored fat and promote the storage of glucose as fat. This implies that your body finds it more difficult to retrieve and burn fat that has been stored as fuel when insulin levels are high, which can cause an increase in weight or make the goal of losing weight rigorous to achieve.

3. Control of Appetite: Insulin affects fullness and appetite as well. Growing insulin levels after a meal can help you feel fuller by informing your brain that you have eaten enough. This information pathway, however, may be thrown off in insulin-resistant people, which could result in binging and eventual addition of weight.

Seven Ways of Controlling Blood Sugar to Lose Weight

Adopting a comprehensive strategy that incorporates food and lifestyle treatments is essential to controlling insulin and blood sugar levels to achieve the goal of losing weight and enjoying better health. Here are seven tactics to think about:

1. Emphasize Whole Foods: Place a strong emphasis on nutrient-dense, whole foods like fruits, vegetables, lean meats, healthy fats, and complex carbohydrates (like whole grains and legumes). In contrast to refined carbohydrates and processed foods, these foods have a lower glycemic index meaning that they have a lower effect on the blood sugar level, which results in slower and more consistent spikes in blood sugar.

2. Balance Macronutrients: Make sure that each meal contains a healthy proportion of fats, proteins, and carbohydrates. By consuming carbohydrates with protein and good fats, the assimilation of sugar into the blood can be slowed down and insulin surges can be avoided.

3. Select Low-Glycemic Options: When ingesting carbohydrates, steer clear of high-glycemic items like white bread, sugary snacks, and sweetened beverages in favor of low-glycemic items like sweet potatoes, quinoa, and legumes. Insulin and blood sugar levels increase more gradually after eating low-glycemic foods.

4. Exercise Portion Control: Pay attention to how much you eat to prevent overindulging your body with calories and carbs, which can cause insulin and blood sugar to rise.

5. Consistent Exercise: Include consistent exercise in your regimen to help enhance insulin sensitivity, which enables cells to respond to insulin and control blood sugar levels more effectively. Strength training and cardiovascular exercises (like cycling and brisk walking) are both advantageous.

6. Control Stress: Prolonged stress can lead to insulin resistance and inhibit the adequate control of blood sugar. It's important to include stress-relieving activities like yoga, deep breathing techniques, mindfulness meditation, and relaxing pastimes.

7. Get Enough Sleep: Make getting enough sleep a priority. Not getting enough sleep can cause insulin and other hormone levels to fluctuate, which can lead to an increase in weight and metabolic problems.

A healthy control of blood sugar and insulin function is critical for effective weight control and hormonal balance. You can support these functions by implementing a balanced approach that prioritizes eating wholesome foods, exercising, reducing stress, and getting enough sleep.

CHAPTER THREE

The Effect of Thyroid Hormones on Weight Control

The thyroid gland is essential for controlling the body's metabolism, production of energy, and general hormonal balance. The addition of weight or difficulties in losing weight are among the results that can arise from the thyroid not working at its best. This chapter will examine the relationship between metabolism, thyroid health, and methods for enhancing thyroid function to promote the aim of losing weight and better health.

Mastering the Relationship Between Metabolism and Thyroid Hormones in Weight Loss

Thyroxine (T4) and triiodothyronine (T3) are the two main hormones that the thyroid gland produces and are crucial for controlling metabolism. The pace at which the body breaks down food into energy is known as the metabolic rate, and it is mostly regulated by these hormones. Metabolism runs smoothly when thyroid hormone levels are in harmony and operating normally, which supports healthy weight control.

On the other hand, a number of variables might interfere with thyroid function, which can result in a lack of hormone harmony and metabolic problems. Typical thyroid conditions include hyperthyroidism, in which the thyroid generates an excess of hormones, and hypothyroidism, in which the thyroid produces inadequate amounts of hormones. Both disorders may affect metabolism and exacerbate problems associated with body weight.

Evidence of hypothyroidism frequently includes constipation, dry skin, hair loss, lethargy, and weight gain. On the other hand, indications of hyperthyroidism include increased appetite, anxiety, sleeplessness, rapid heartbeat, and weight loss. The complex interplay between thyroid hormones and metabolism is brought to light by these abnormalities.

Seven Methods to Enhance Thyroid Function

Maintaining general health and controlling weight depends on thyroid function. The following seven techniques can help to maximize thyroid function:

1. Diet Rich in Nutrients: Eating a well-balanced diet full of vital nutrients is important for thyroid function. Incorporate meals rich in zinc, vitamin D, iodine, and selenium since these nutrients are essential for the synthesis and operation of thyroid hormones. These nutrients can be obtained from leafy greens, dairy products, nuts, and seeds.

2. Control Stress: Prolonged stress can interfere with hormone balance and thyroid function. Try stress-relieving methods like yoga, deep breathing exercises, meditation, or taking up a fun hobby. Getting enough sleep is also essential for thyroid health support and stress control.

3. Frequent Exercise: Exercise improves general health and metabolism. To increase metabolic rate and promote thyroid function, combine weight training exercises with aerobic exercises like swimming, cycling, or brisk walking. On most days of the week, try to get yourself involved in a minimum of thirty minutes of moderate or aerobic exercise.

4. Steer clear of Toxins: Lack of protection from heavy metals, pollution, and pesticides in the environment can cause thyroid dysfunction. Reduce your

subjection to these pollutants by filtering your drinking water, buying unprocessed products, and using chemical-free cleaning supplies.

5. Watch Your Iodine Intake: Although iodine is necessary for thyroid function, too much of it can be harmful, particularly for those who already have thyroid issues. To find your ideal iodine intake, speak with a healthcare provider. If necessary, take into account iodine-rich meals or supplements.

6. Supportive Supplements: Apart from iodine and selenium, some supplements can also assist thyroid function. These supplements consist of vitamin D, omega-3 fatty acids, and adaptogenic herbs such as rhodiola and ashwagandha. Nevertheless, before beginning any new supplement regimen, it's important to get medical advice.

7. Thyroid Testing: To keep watch on thyroid health and identify any lack of harmony early on, consistent thyroid function testing, including TSH (thyroid-stimulating hormone), T4, and T3 levels, is recommended. Determine thyroid function in close collaboration with your healthcare professional, and modify therapy or lifestyle choices as necessary.

You can enhance weight control and general health by adopting these lifestyle strategies, which can aid normal thyroid function, optimize metabolism, and encourage general hormone harmony.

Finally, general hormone harmony and metabolism are closely related to thyroid health. You may improve thyroid function and greatly assist your body to lose weight by putting an emphasis on nutrient-rich foods, controlling stress, getting consistent exercise, avoiding toxins, taking the right amount of iodine, taking supportive supplements, and having frequent thyroid tests. Collaborating with medical specialists is essential to creating a customized strategy that targets your unique thyroid requirements and wellness objectives.

CHAPTER FOUR

The Effect of Nutrition on Hormone Balance for Weight Loss

Nutrition is a key component in the pursuit of regulating hormones for the purpose of losing weight and staying in good health. Our hormonal health is strongly impacted by the food we eat; it affects everything from energy levels and metabolic rate to emotional state and desires. We may improve our nutrition to assist hormonal balance by concentrating on foods that support hormones and planning our meals methodically.

Understanding how eating affects hormones is vital before delving into certain foods and meal plans. Hormones are message-sending chemicals in the body that control appetite, fullness, emotional state, metabolic rate, and other body processes. While some foods are essential for the synthesis of hormones, others that are taken in excess or insufficiently can upset the balance of hormones.

Seven Various Foods That Support Hormone Balance

1. Healthy Fats: They provide essential fatty acids that help to facilitate hormone synthesis, particularly estrogen and testosterone. It's important for you to include foods like avocados, almonds, seeds, and olive oil that are rich in healthy fats in your diet.

2. Omega-3 Fatty Acids: They assist in improving the ability of hormones to convey information, as well as in lowering inflammation. It's important for you to

include foods like walnuts, flaxseeds, chia seeds, and fatty fish like salmon that are rich in omega-3 fatty acids in your diet.

3. Protein: They are required for the production of hormones and for maintaining muscle mass, both of which are critical for a healthy metabolism. It's important for you to include foods like lentils, beans, fish, fowl, and tofu that are rich in lean protein in your diet.

4. Fiber-rich foods: In addition to helping with digestion and blood sugar regulation, fiber also increases satiety and reduces the risk of insulin spikes, which can upset hormone balance. In order to maximize your intake of fiber, eat an abundance of fruits, vegetables, whole grains, and legumes.

5. Antioxidant-Rich Foods: They contain antioxidants that help to prevent oxidative stress and maintain hormonal balance in general. It's important for you to eat a variety of vibrant fruits and vegetables, such as broccoli, spinach, kale, and berries that are rich in antioxidants.

6. Probiotic Foods: They enhance gut health, which establishes hormone harmony and helps the immune system to function better. They include fermented foods such as kimchi, kefir, yogurt, and sauerkraut.

7. Herbs and Spices: Like omega-3 fatty acids, herbs and spices contain components that help to lower inflammation, and also assist in regulating hormone function. It's important for you to add seasonings like garlic, ginger, turmeric, and cinnamon to your diet to obtain these herbal substances.

Seven Essential Rules for Hormone Balance Meal Planning

For weight loss and hormonal balance to be supported, a balanced diet plan must be developed. Here's how to arrange your meals for the best possible hormone health:

1. Balanced Macronutrients: Macronutrients include fats, proteins, and carbohydrates. It's important for you to try to have the right amounts of healthy fats, protein, and carbohydrates at every meal. This equilibrium promotes the synthesis of hormones and aids in controlling blood sugar levels.

2. Maintain a Consistent Eating Schedule: To control hormones that are associated with hunger such as ghrelin and leptin, maintain a consistent meal schedule. Steer clear of prolonged fasts since they may upset the hormonal balance.

3. Portion Control: Manage your portions to avoid overindulging, which can result in a lack of hormone harmony and insulin resistance. Dish your meals with smaller plates and pay attention to your body's signals of satiety and starvation.

4. Hydration: Endeavor to drink lots of water to stay hydrated all through the day. Metabolic rate and the activities of hormones can be negatively impacted by dehydration.

5. Incorporate Hormone-Supportive Foods: Make an effort to frequently include the previously stated hormone-supportive foods in your meals and refreshments.

6. Reduce Processed Foods: Refined carbohydrates, sugary refreshments, and processed foods should all be avoided because they can cause hormone swings and insulin resistance.

7. Mindful Eating: Engage in mindful eating by chewing carefully, concentrating on your meal, and being aware of your body's signals of starvation and satiation. In addition to promoting good digestion, this can stop binging.

You may fuel your body, promote hormonal harmony, and work toward the goal of losing weight in a sustainable manner by including foods that assist hormone harmony in your diet and adhering to a comprehensive meal plan. Endeavor to constantly pay attention to your body's signals, maintain a regular diet, and ask medical specialists or nutritionists for advice when necessary.

CHAPTER FIVE

The Influence of Exercise on Hormone Balance for Weight Loss

Exercise is essential for the purpose of achieving hormone harmony and losing weight. Exercise and hormone control has a complex and multidimensional interaction, with various kinds and magnitudes of exercise having an influence on different hormones. By comprehending this active interaction, people can better create exercise regimens that enhance hormone harmony and help them achieve their goal of losing weight.

Exercise's Effect on Six Essential Hormones for Weight Loss

Exercise has a significant impact on balancing hormones for weight loss, influencing important hormones related to metabolism, hunger regulation, and general health. The following are six of the main hormones that exercise affects:

1. Insulin: Exercise increases insulin responsiveness, which makes it possible for cells to assimilate glucose from the bloodstream more efficiently. This assists in balancing blood sugar levels and lowers the chance of developing insulin resistance, a disease linked to metabolic problems and the addition of weight.

2. Cortisol: Exercise is known to trigger the discharge of cortisol, which is commonly known as the 'stress hormone'. Moderate exercise assists in controlling the release of cortisol hormone, enabling a healthy stress response, though

persistently increased cortisol levels can lead to metabolic disruptions and the addition of weight.

3. Growth Hormone: Vigorous exercise, especially high-intensity interval training (HIIT) and strength training increases the release of growth hormone. Growth of muscles, breaking down of fat, and general metabolic processes are all significantly impacted by growth hormones.

4. Adrenaline and Norepinephrine: These hormones are also known as 'fight-or-flight' hormones. They increase the process of exercise, releasing stored energy and speeding up the metabolic rate, thereby aiding in weight loss. Additionally, they support the 'Excess Post-Exercise Oxygen Consumption (EPOC)', a situation in which the body continues to burn calories at an increased rate after exercise.

5. Leptin and Ghrelin: The starvation hormone, ghrelin, promotes appetite while the fullness hormone, leptin, reduces appetite. Frequent exercise promotes feelings of fullness and decreases binging by balancing these hormones, thereby aiding in weight loss.

6. Endorphins: Exercise causes the discharge of endorphins, which are natural morphine-like substances that enhance pleasure and lessen the experience of pain. This can improve motivation, mood, and general comfort — all of which are important for maintaining enduring fitness routines, thereby aiding in weight loss.

Six Crucial Pointers for Creating a Hormone-Balancing Exercise Program

A hormone-balancing exercise program should incorporate a range of exercises that focus on various hormone responses and physiological systems. Here are six essential ideas to assist you in planning a quality hormone-balancing exercise program:

1. Incorporate Strength Training: To promote the production of growth hormone, increase lean muscle mass, and speed up metabolic rate for weight loss, strength training including weightlifting, bodyweight exercises, and resistance band workouts is crucial. Endeavor to do between two to three sessions of strength training every week.

2. Include High-Intensity Interval Training (HIIT): HIIT entails brief intervals of high-intensity training interspersed with rest or reduced-intensity intervals. This kind of exercise increases the discharge of hormones such as norepinephrine and adrenaline, burns fat more effectively, and strengthens cardiovascular fitness. Endeavor to do between one to two sessions of HIIT every week.

3. Include Aerobic Exercise: Exercises that increase heart rate, and endurance, and assist in controlling weight are known as aerobic exercise. Some examples of aerobic exercise are riding, brisk walking, swimming, dancing, and cycling. Endeavor to do a minimum of three to five days of moderate-to-intense aerobic exercise every week. It's advisable to do longer or more intense sessions, depending on your level of fitness.

4. Incorporate Flexibility and Mobility Work: Yoga, stretches, and mobility drills help to increase the range of motion in the joints, ease tense muscles, and enhance flexibility. Engaging in these activities can improve recuperation, reduce the risk of injury, and promote general physical health.

5. Make Rest and Recovery a Priority: Hormone harmony and the ability to exercise in general depend on getting enough sleep and recovering from injuries. Make sure your training plan includes rest days, give adequate sleep a high priority, and engage in stress-relieving techniques like deep breathing or meditation.

6. Listen to Your Body: Focus on the cues your body gives you and modify the time and magnitude of your workouts in accordance with those cues. Maintain an exercise proportion that permits advancement while honoring your body's need for recuperation. Exercising in excess might result in a lack of hormone harmony, exhaustion, and an elevated likelihood of injury that could put the entire process of exercise to a halt.

You may design a hormone-balancing exercise program that assists in achieving the goal of losing weight, improves metabolic function, and fosters general health and comfort by implementing these ideas into your workout routine. Achieving long-lasting benefits requires careful attention to your body's reactions, consistency, and variation.

Finally, exercise is essential for balancing hormones for weight loss since it affects important hormones related to metabolic rate, hunger regulation, and general health. Individuals can enable themselves to achieve the goal of losing weight by promoting hormone harmony through the establishment of a balanced fitness regimen that includes strength training, high-intensity interval training (HIIT), aerobic exercise, flexibility workout, and enough rest.

CHAPTER SIX

Enhancing Hormone Harmony for Weight Loss by Controlling Stress

Stress has become a menace in our present fast-paced universe, having an impact on our mental, emotional, and physical health. Stress is a major factor in hormone harmony and weight control, particularly with regard to the hormone that is called cortisol. This chapter will examine the complex connection between stress, cortisol, and weight control. It will also cover practical stress-reduction methods that help achieve hormone harmony.

The adrenal glands release cortisol, sometimes known as the 'stress hormone', in reaction to any kind of stress, be it psychological, emotional, or physical. Cortisol has certain advantages when released in moderation; it helps control inflammation, blood sugar, and metabolism. On the other hand, long-term stress can raise cortisol levels, which can negatively impact weight control and hormonal harmony.

Six Negative Consequences of High Cortisol Hormone Levels As A Result of Stress

1. A greater desire and hunger, particularly for sweet and high-calorie foods.

2. The buildup of fat, especially visceral fat in the abdomen.

3. A slower metabolic rate and use of energy.

4. Reduced insulin responsiveness, which results in hyperglycemia.

5. Disintegration of muscle cells and decreased muscular mass.

6. Obstruction of other hormones, like ghrelin and leptin, that regulate weight via the control of appetite for food.

Consequently, extended subjection to elevated cortisol levels may result in the accumulation of excess fat, particularly in the abdominal region, which has been connected to a number of health problems, including type-2 diabetes and cardiovascular disease.

Eight Effective Strategies for Controlling Stress to Achieve Hormone Balance for Weight Loss

It is imperative that you include stress-relief practices into your daily habits in order to promote the attainment of hormone harmony and weight control. These methods support resilience and general health in addition to reducing cortisol levels. Here are eight successful tactics:

1. Mindfulness Meditation: To develop the awareness of the here-and-now and lessen stress susceptibility, exercise mindfulness meditation. Every day, set aside some time to concentrate on your breath, your thoughts, and your body's feelings without passing judgment.

2. Exercise: Frequent exercise helps to stabilize the levels of cortisol in the body, acting as a potent stress reliever. For the purpose of boosting general wellness and resilience, try to incorporate strength training with aerobic activities (such as brisk walking, dancing, or swimming).

3. Deep Breathing Exercises: To enable the body to get into the mood of relaxation and reduce cortisol levels, engage in deep breathing exercises like diaphragmatic breathing or box breathing. Inhale slowly and deeply, making sure to release all of the air.

4. Yoga and Tai Chi: Make an effort to include these mind-body exercises into your regimen. They help to maintain hormone harmony and lower stress by combining movement, breathwork, and mindfulness.

5. Sufficient Sleep: To help with hormone balance and lower cortisol levels, make sleep a priority. Establish a calming bedtime ritual and make the most of your sleeping environment to achieve between seven to nine hours of peaceful sleep every night.

6. Social Support: To assist one another with knowledge, get emotional backing, and create a feeling of community that helps reduce stress, and keep up strong social ties with friends, family, or support groups.

7. Time Management: To lessen overload and avoid long-term stress, set priorities for your chores and arrange your tasks properly. If possible, assign tasks to others and get comfortable declining unimportant assignments.

8. Healthy Nutrition: Nutrient-dense foods such as fruits, vegetables, whole grains, lean meats, and healthy fats should make up a balanced diet. Steer clear of processed meals, sugar, and excess caffeine as these can result in stress, causing a lack of hormone harmony that will make it difficult to lose weight.

By adopting these stress-reduction methods into your daily routine, you may assist your body in losing weight, successfully controlling cortisol levels, and establishing hormonal balance. Always keep in mind that finding balance requires persistence and time, so practice self-compassion and patience along the way.

CHAPTER SEVEN

Utilizing Herbal Remedies for Balancing Hormones for Weight Loss

Achieving hormone harmony is essential for weight loss and general health. Our bodies use hormones as mediators to control a number of processes, such as energy levels, hunger, and metabolism. Hormone imbalances can cause mood changes, dullness, an increase in weight, and other health problems. Herbal treatments provide a safe, all-natural method of promoting hormonal balance, even in addition to medical procedures. This chapter will cover a variety of herbs that are well-known for helping with weight reduction and for balancing hormones.

Five Different Herbs That Can Assist in Hormone Balance

1. Ashwagandha (Withania somnifera): Used extensively in Ayurvedic medicine, ashwagandha is a performance-enhancing herb. It aids in the regulation of cortisol levels, which are the main stress hormone and which, when increased, can cause an increase in weight, particularly in the abdominal region. Ashwagandha supports hormone balance, which is necessary for a healthy metabolic rate and effective weight control, by lowering stress and enhancing adrenal function.

2. Maca (Lepidium meyenii): This Andean native's root is well-known for promoting hormone harmony, especially in women. It aids in the control of estrogen levels, which is advantageous for women going through menopause or having irregular menstruation. General comfort and a healthier weight are enhanced by well-regulated estrogen levels.

3. Licorice Root (Glycyrrhiza glabra): This herb is useful for treating stress and adrenal exhaustion because it contains substances that resemble cortisol's effects. Licorice root helps preserve hormone harmony and inhibits cortisol-induced weight gain by promoting adrenal function. But, it's crucial to consume licorice root sparingly and under medical supervision, particularly for people with high blood pressure or other medical issues.

4. Vitex (Vitex agnus-castus): This herb, which is sometimes referred to as chasteberry, is a well-liked herb for women's health, especially when it comes to hormonal abnormalities associated with the menstrual cycle. It supports progesterone balance and aids in luteinizing hormone regulation, which may help women who experience irregular menstruation, premenstrual syndrome, or reproductive problems. It follows that as Vitex herbs help in establishing hormone balance, it indirectly promotes a healthy weight and efficient metabolism.

5. Rhodiola (Rhodiola rosea): Rhodiola is a performance-enhancing herb that promotes adrenal function and aids in the body's adjustment to stress. Rhodiola assists in establishing hormone harmony in the body, and it can help with weight control by lowering stress-related cortisol levels. This is especially beneficial for people who have stress-induced cravings for food.

Five Various Herbal Supplements to Help Lose Weight

1. Green Tea Extract: Abounding in antioxidants called catechins, green tea promotes fat oxidation and breakdown. By boosting thermogenesis — the process of burning calories to produce heat — and raising energy exertion, green tea extract supplements can help with the achievement of the goal of losing weight.

2. Fenugreek (Trigonella foenum-graecum): Abounding in soluble fiber, fenugreek seeds aid in controlling blood sugar and encourage fullness. This herbal supplement can assist an individual in maintaining a healthy metabolic rate and

losing weight by lowering the rate of digestion and increasing the responsiveness of the body cells to insulin.

3. Garcinia Cambogia: Hydroxycitric acid is found in the tropical fruit Garcinia cambogia, which has been shown to suppress hunger and prevent the formation of fat. Despite the fact that there is conflicting evidence on the efficacy of garcinia cambogia supplements, several studies do indicate that they may help with a satisfactory decrease in weight when supported with exercise and a proper diet.

4. Cinnamon: In addition to being a tasty spice, cinnamon may help with the goal of losing weight. It assists in controlling the blood sugar levels of the body, which is essential in avoiding insulin surges that may result in fat storage. Including cinnamon in your diet or taking supplements may help promote proper control of blood sugar and metabolic rate, which is important for achieving the goal of losing weight.

5. Turmeric (Curcuma longa): Turmeric contains a chemical substance known as curcumin, which possesses reasonable anti-inflammatory and antioxidant properties, assisting with the achievement of the goal of losing weight. It aids in reducing inflammation, which is connected to metabolic diseases and obesity. Including turmeric in your food or taking pills can help your body's metabolism and general wellness.

It's crucial to remember that although herbal medicines offer potential benefits, each person may respond differently, so speaking with a healthcare provider is advised — especially if you have hidden medical concerns or are taking medication. The usefulness of these herbs and supplements in establishing hormone harmony and assisting with the achievement of the goal of losing weight can be increased by incorporating them within a comprehensive approach that also includes consistent exercise, a proper diet, stress control, and enough sleep.

<h1 style="text-align:center">CHAPTER EIGHT</h1>

Mastering Hormone Replacement Therapy For Weight Loss

Hormone Replacement Therapy (HRT) is becoming a very useful technique in the field of hormone balance and weight control. This chapter explores the many facets of hormone replacement therapy (HRT), covering topics such as common hormone replacement therapy options, advantages of hormone replacement therapy, and disadvantages of hormone replacement therapy.

Five Common Hormone Replacement Therapy Options

In hormone replacement therapy, the body's original hormones are supplemented or replaced with artificial or bioidentical hormones. These hormones may consist of thyroid hormones, progesterone, testosterone, estrogen, and other hormones. Restoring hormone balance, reducing symptoms associated with lack of harmony, and enhancing general health are the objectives of hormone replacement therapy.

1. Estrogen Replacement Therapy (ERT): Women who suffer from menopausal symptoms like mood swings, vaginal dryness, hot flashes, and night sweats are frequently recommended estrogen replacement therapy. It can be applied topically as creams, tablets, vaginal rings, and patches.

2. Progesterone Replacement Therapy: To safeguard the uterus and lower the danger of a precancerous state in which there is an uneven thickening of the uterine wall, progesterone is frequently taken in conjunction with estrogen. It can be administered intrauterinally (IUDs), orally, or topically.

3. Testosterone Replacement Therapy (TRT): TRT is mostly used to treat an abnormally decreased levels of testosterone in men, which can cause weariness, obesity, diminished muscular mass, and reduced libido. It can be applied as implants, gels, patches, or injections.

4. Thyroid Hormone Replacement: People with hypothyroidism, a disorder marked by hypoactive thyroid gland, are administered thyroid hormone replacement. Levothyroxine is one of the artificial thyroid hormones that are applied to get the thyroid and metabolism back to normal.

5. Bioidentical Hormone Replacement Therapy (BHRT): This is all about the application of foreign hormones that are structurally similar to those produced by the body. These hormones are thought to have less adverse effects than artificial hormones because they are frequently sourced from plant sources.

Five Common Advantages of Hormone Replacement Therapy

1. Symptom Relief: Lack of hormone harmony symptoms like hot flushes, emotional instabilities, exhaustion, and sleeplessness can be successfully treated with hormone replacement therapy.

2. Better Quality of Life: Hormone replacement therapy (HRT) can improve emotional stability, cognitive performance, general health, and total hormone harmony.

3. Bone Health: In postmenopausal women, estrogen replacement therapy can assist in preserving the density of bones and lowering the chances of fractures and osteoporosis.

4. Libido and Sexual Function: Hormone replacement therapy, specifically estrogen therapy for females and testosterone therapy for males, can assist in enhancing sexual capacity and desires, especially in the elderly.

5. Metabolic Effects: Hormone relacement therapy may help enhance lipid profiles, insulin responsiveness, and weight control, among other aspects of metabolic health.

Five Common Disadvantages of Hormone Replacement Therapy

1. Side Effects: Gaining weight, breast soreness, mood fluctuations, headaches, and a feeling of vomiting are a few of the side effects of hormone replacement therapy.

2. Enhanced Risk of Blood Clots: Estrogen replacement therapy may increase the danger of blood clots, stroke, and heart disease, particularly when paired with specific risk factors.

3. Risk of Breast Cancer: The link between lasting estrogen-progestin therapy and a higher risk of breast cancer is still up for discussion.

4. Endometrial Hyperplasia: In women without uteruses, unrestricted estrogen therapy can result in a precancerous state where in the lining of the uterine space thickens unevenly, known as endometrial hyperplasia.

5. Individual Variability: Because people react to hormone replacement therapy differently, it may be necessary to carefully examine and modify the dosage and formulation in order to get the desired results.

Finally, hormone replacement therapy is a useful strategy for reestablishing hormonal balance and treating a range of medical issues, including weight control. To customize treatment regimens, it is crucial to balance the dangers and potential advantages and to collaborate closely with medical professionals. Making the most of the advantages of hormone replacement therapy while reducing any potential risks requires knowledge of available options, personalized consideration of circumstances, and consistent follow-ups.

CONCLUSION

This book has explored the complex relationship between hormones and controlling weight, offering helpful tips and methods that are especially suited to women. We have discovered the critical role lack of hormone harmony plays in influencing variations in weight and general health through a thorough investigation of these imbalances.

Recapitulating the main tactics covered in this short book, we have stressed the significance of adopting a holistic strategy that includes proper nutrition, exercise, stress reduction, and commensurate sleep. Women can assist their bodies to achieve hormone balance and encourage enduring weight loss by consuming a nutrient-dense, whole foods-based diet high in fiber, protein, healthy fats, and critical nutrients. To achieve hormonal balance, it is equally important to prioritize restful sleep, practice stress-reduction strategies like mindfulness and meditation, and engage in consistent exercise.

As you proceed on your path to achieving hormone balance, keep in mind that patience and consistency are key components. It takes time to treat and readjust hormonal imbalances, so you must approach the goal with a long-term perspective. Remain dedicated to putting the techniques in this book into practice, pay attention to your body's signals, and get expert help when required.

Fundamentally, women can open the door to long-term weight loss and enhanced general health and comfort by promoting hormone harmony through lifestyle adjustments and customized tactics. I wish you strength, energy, and enduring success on your path to hormonal balance.

ABOUT THE AUTHOR

James Edwards is a unique writer of numerous short books. His specialty is penning nonfiction publications that have the power to favorably influence readers' lives on the subjects they cover. James takes a perceptive approach to writing that blends useful techniques with deep understandings discovered via diligent study of the subject matter.

"FINANCIAL LITERACY FOR TEENS AND YOUNG ADULTS" is one of his best-selling books. Other bestsellers include "UNDERSTANDING MEDICAL TERMINOLOGY BY MASTERING PREFIX AND SUFFIX," "LOWER CHOLESTEROL NATURALLY," and "A SHORT DESCRIPTION OF THE SECRET OF RELIEVING PAIN BY TRAINING YOUR NERVOUS SYSTEM DIFFERENTLY." He is a prolific author of other short nonfiction books. Every word James writes is infused with his genuine desire to positively impact every reader's life and his passion for personal progress.

Start reading James Edwards's books now to begin your road toward a more purposeful and happy existence.

You can discover his other useful and highly interesting short books by visiting his author central page here: https://www.amazon.com/author/jamesedwards1974

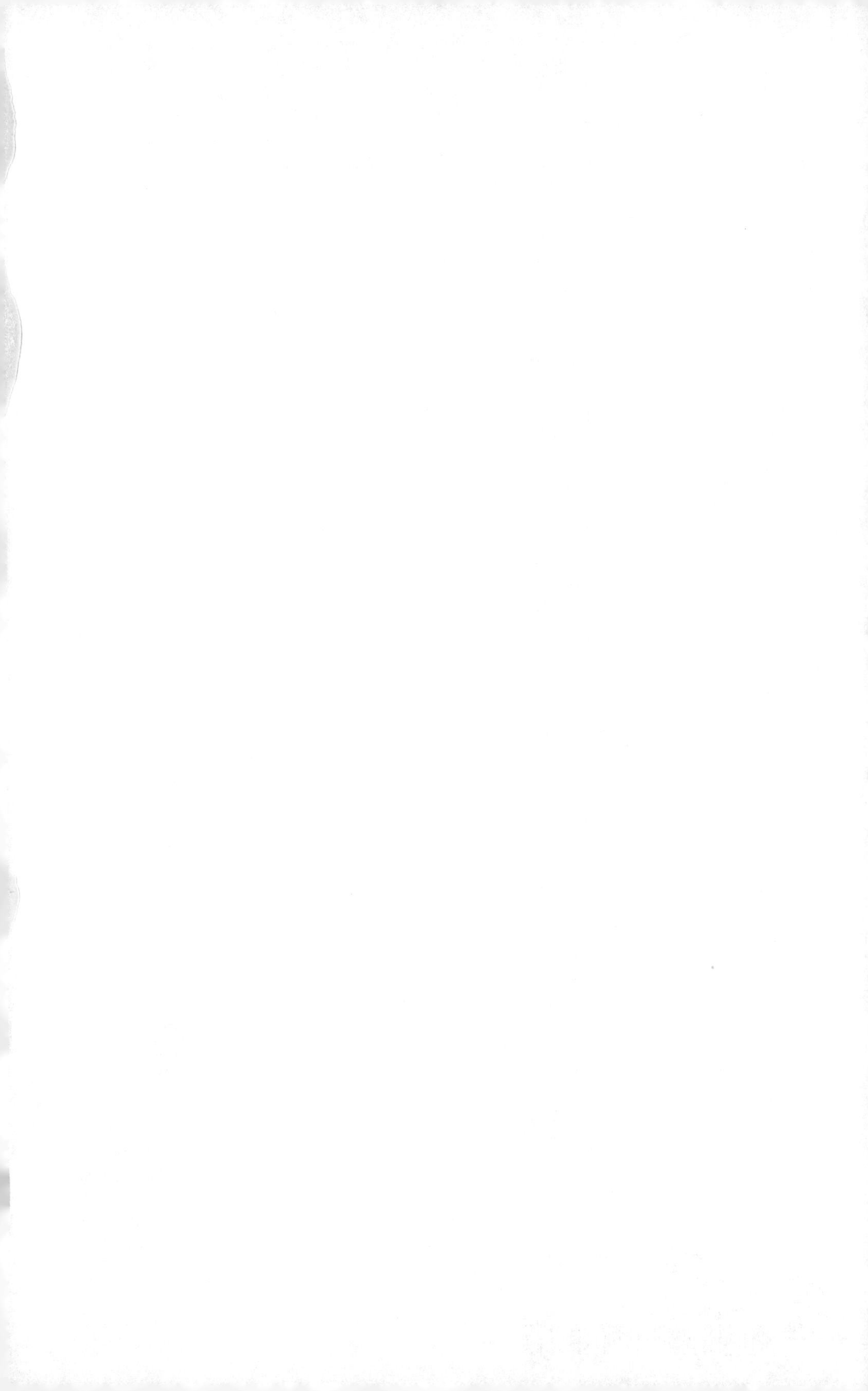

www.ingramcontent.com/pod-product-compliance
Lightning Source LLC
Chambersburg PA
CBHW072342270726
48659CB00023B/2309